HEALTHY AGING THROUGH JUICING AND SMOOTHIES

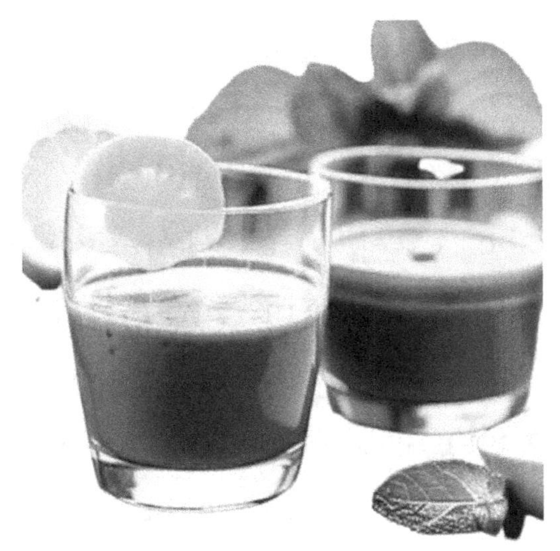

A 62-Day Program for Men Over 60

Michael S. Owen

TABLE OF CONTENT

INTRODUCTION

My friend's father had recently turned sixty-two and his health was not at its best. He had started to experience a number of aches and pains and his energy levels were low. I was worried about him and wanted to help, so I decided to talk to my friend so I can educate him about the importance of healthy aging and how juicing and smoothies could help.

I gave him a copy of this book "Healthy Aging through Juicing and Smoothies: A 62-Day Program for Men over 60" and showed him the benefits of juicing and smoothies for healthy aging. I also explained to him the nutritional benefits of juicing and smoothies, as well as their positive effects on gut, heart, brain and immune health

We discussed the 62-day healthy aging program described in the book and he agreed to try it. We started by having him take a few days to get used to the idea of juicing and smoothies and to prepare the ingredients.

He then began the program and was amazed at how quickly his energy levels increased and how his aches and pains began to subside. He also found the delicious recipes for juicing and smoothies in this book to be easy to make and very enjoyable. He started creating his own unique combinations and experimenting with different flavors. After completing the program, he felt much better and had more energy than he had in a long time.

He was so grateful for the knowledge I had shared with him and the positive changes it had made in his life. He now believes that juicing and smoothies are essential to healthy aging and recommends them to everyone he meets. Even at the end of the program he continued with juicing and smoothies.

What is Healthy Aging?

What is Healthy Aging? Healthy aging is the process of maintaining good physical, mental, and emotional health as we age. It involves making lifestyle changes that can reduce the risk of chronic diseases and other age-related illnesses. Healthy aging also involves finding ways to stay active, engaged, and connected with others.

The key to healthy aging is to maintain a balanced diet, get plenty of exercise, and manage stress. Eating a balanced diet that includes fruits, vegetables, whole grains, and lean proteins can help ensure you get the nutrients you need for optimal health.

Regular exercise helps to strengthen bones and muscles, improve balance, and reduce symptoms of depression and anxiety. And managing stress through relaxation techniques, such as **yoga, tai chi,** and **meditation,** can help keep your body and mind in balance. In addition to diet and exercise, there are other ways to support healthy aging.

These include getting **regular check-ups, avoiding smoking, limiting alcohol intake, and staying socially connected.** All of these steps can help you maintain optimal health as you age.

Understanding the Aging Process

Aging is a natural process that begins in early adulthood and continues throughout our lives. As we get older, our bodies and minds undergo changes. Physical changes can include wrinkles and gray hair, vision and hearing loss, decreased mobility and muscle strength, and a decrease in energy levels.

Mental changes can include a decrease in short-term memory and an increase in forgetfulness. These changes can be difficult to accept and cope with, but understanding the aging process can help you make lifestyle changes that will support your overall health and wellbeing. It's important to remember that aging is a normal part of life and that everyone goes through it. By understanding the aging process, you can find ways to stay healthy and active as you age.

All of these steps can help you maintain optimal health as you age. This book also outlines a 62-day healthy aging program that provides step-by-step instructions on how to incorporate juicing and smoothies into your daily routine. This program includes guidelines on which ingredients to use, how to prepare and drink the juices and smoothies, and tips on how to make sure you get the most out of them. It also includes a variety of delicious recipes that are easy to make and enjoyable to drink. Following this program can help men over sixty achieve optimal health and wellbeing.

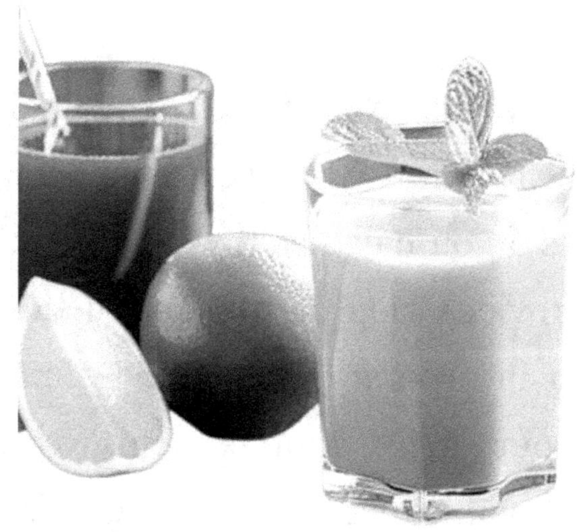

CHAPTER ONE

BENEFITS OF JUICING AND SMOOTHIES

The Benefits of Juicing and Smoothies for Healthy Aging

Juicing and smoothies can have many benefits for healthy aging. Juicing and smoothies provide concentrated sources of essential vitamins and minerals, which can help support overall health and wellbeing.

They are also high in antioxidants, which can help to protect cells from damage caused by free radicals. In addition, juicing and smoothies can help support gut health, as they provide beneficial probiotics, prebiotics, and fiber that can help keep the digestive system functioning properly. They can also help support heart health by providing essential vitamins and minerals that can help protect against heart disease. Juicing and smoothies can also help support **brain health** by providing nutrients that can help protect against neuron damage and reduce the risk of dementia.

Finally, juicing and smoothies can help support immune health by providing essential vitamins and minerals that can help strengthen the immune system.

The importance of Juicing and Smoothies for Gut Health

Juicing and smoothies are important for gut health, as they provide beneficial probiotics, prebiotics, and fiber that can help keep the digestive system functioning properly. Probiotics are beneficial bacteria that can help promote a healthy balance of gut flora, while prebiotics are non-digestible fibers that can help feed the probiotics. Both of these can help support a healthy digestive system.

In addition, fiber from fruits and vegetables can help keep the digestive system functioning properly. It can help to keep the bowels regular and reduce the risk of constipation. Fiber can also help reduce the risk of certain diseases, such as colon cancer and diverticulitis. The vitamins and minerals found in juices and smoothies can help to support **gut health** by providing essential nutrients that can help protect against infections and reduce inflammation.

The importance of Juicing and Smoothies for Heart Health

Juicing and smoothies are important for heart health, as they provide essential vitamins and minerals that can help protect against heart disease. Fruits and vegetables are high in fiber, which can help reduce cholesterol levels and reduce the risk of heart disease. They are also high in antioxidants, which can help reduce inflammation and protect against cell damage.

In addition, juicing and smoothies can provide essential vitamins and minerals, such as **vitamins B6 and B12, folate, magnesium, and potassium.** These vitamins and minerals can help reduce the risk of heart disease by supporting healthy blood pressure and cholesterol levels. Finally, juicing and smoothies can provide essential fatty acids, such as **omega-3 fatty acids,** which can help reduce inflammation and support heart health.

How juicing and smoothies can improve the Brain Health

Juicing and smoothies can help improve brain health by providing essential vitamins and minerals that can help protect against **neuron damage** and reduce the risk of **dementia.** Fruits and vegetables are high in **antioxidants,** which can help reduce inflammation and protect against cell damage. They are also high in **omega-3 fatty acids,** which can help reduce inflammation and support brain health. It can also provide essential vitamins and minerals, such as **vitamin B12, folate, magnesium, and potassium.**

These vitamins and minerals can help improve **cognitive function**, reduce the risk of **stroke, and reduce the risk of dementia.** It can also provide essential fatty acids, such as omega-3 fatty acids, which can help reduce inflammation and support brain health.

How Juicing and Smoothies can improve Immune Health

Juicing and smoothies can help improve immune health by providing essential vitamins and minerals that can help strengthen the immune system. Fruits and vegetables are high in antioxidants, which can help reduce inflammation and protect against cell damage.

They are also high in vitamins **A, C, and E,** which can help to boost the immune system. In addition, juicing and smoothies can provide essential fatty acids, such as **omega-3 fatty acids**, which can help reduce inflammation and support immune health. They can also provide essential vitamins and minerals, such as vitamin **B12,**

folate, magnesium, and potassium, which can help to support a healthy immune system.

Finally, juicing and smoothies can provide beneficial probiotics, prebiotics, and fiber, which can help to support a healthy balance of gut flora and reduce the risk of certain infections.

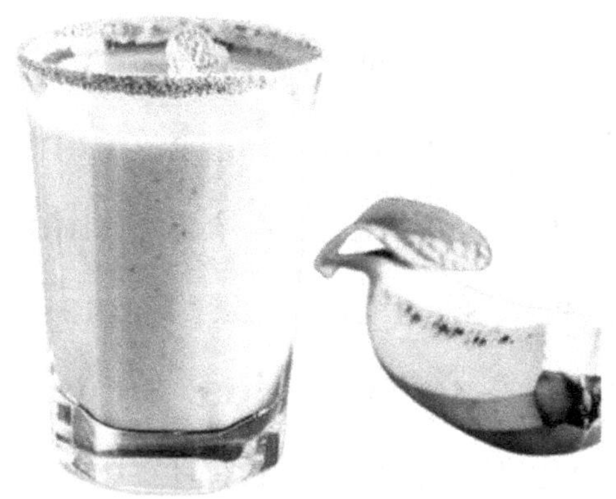

CHAPTER TWO

THE 62-DAY JUICING AND SMOOTHIE PLAN (DAY 1-28)

Day 1-7 smoothies plan for Boosting Energy and Vitality

Day 1: Blueberry-Banana Smoothie

Ingredients:

½ cup blueberries

½ banana

1 cup almond milk

1 teaspoon honey

1 tablespoon flaxseed

Instructions:

- Place the blueberries and banana in a blender.
- Add the almond milk and honey and blend until smooth.
- Add the flaxseed and blend for an additional 30 seconds.
- Pour into a glass and enjoy!

Nutritional Benefits: This smoothie is packed with antioxidants from the blueberries and fiber from the banana, flaxseed, and almond milk. The honey helps to sweeten the smoothie without adding too much sugar, and the flaxseed adds a healthy dose of omega-3 fatty acids.

Day 2: Strawberry-Almond Smoothie

Ingredients:

1 cup strawberries   ¼ cup almonds

1 cup almond milk   1 teaspoon honey

1 teaspoon chia seeds

Instructions:

- Place the strawberries, almonds, and almond milk in a blender.
- Add the honey and chia seeds and blend until smooth.
- Pour into a glass and enjoy!

Nutritional Benefits: This smoothie is packed with antioxidants from the strawberries and healthy fats from the almonds and chia seeds. The honey helps to sweeten the smoothie without adding too much sugar.

Day 3: Pineapple-Coconut Smoothie

Ingredients:

½ cup pineapple   ¼ cup coconut flakes

1 cup coconut milk   1 teaspoon honey

1 teaspoon maca powder

Instructions:

- Place the pineapple, coconut flakes, and coconut milk in a blender.
- Add the honey and maca powder and blend until smooth.
- Pour into a glass and enjoy!

Nutritional Benefits: This smoothie is packed with antioxidants from the pineapple and healthy fats from the coconut flakes and coconut milk. The honey helps to sweeten the smoothie without adding too much sugar, and the maca powder adds a healthy dose of vitamins and minerals.

Day 4: Green Smoothie

Ingredients:

1 cup spinach   ½ banana

½ cup pineapple   1 cup almond milk

1 teaspoon honey   1 teaspoon chia seeds

Instructions:

- Place the spinach, banana, and pineapple in a blender.
- Add the almond milk, honey, and chia seeds and blend until smooth.
- Pour into a glass and enjoy!

Nutritional Benefits: This smoothie is packed with vitamins and minerals from the spinach and fiber from the banana, pineapple, and chia seeds.

Day 5: Mango-Coconut Smoothie

Ingredients:

½ cup mango   ¼ cup coconut flakes

1 cup coconut milk   1 teaspoon honey

1 teaspoon maca powder

Instructions:

- Place the mango, coconut flakes, and coconut milk in a blender.
- Add the honey and maca powder and blend until smooth.
- Pour into a glass and enjoy!

Nutritional Benefits: This smoothie is packed with antioxidants from the mango and healthy fats from the coconut flakes and coconut milk and the maca powder adds a healthy dose of vitamins and minerals.

Day 6: Acai-Cherry Smoothie

Ingredients:

½ cup acai berries	½ cup cherries
1 cup almond milk	1 teaspoon honey
1 tablespoon flaxseed	

Instructions:

- Place the acai berries and cherries in a blender.
- Add the almond milk and honey and blend until smooth.
- Add the flaxseed and blend for an additional 30 seconds.
- Pour into a glass and enjoy!

Nutritional Benefits: This smoothie is packed with antioxidants from the acai berries and cherries and fiber from the flaxseed and almond milk and the flaxseed adds a healthy dose of omega-3 fatty acids.

Day 7: Blueberry-Almond Smoothie

Ingredients:

½ cup blueberries

¼ cup almonds

1 cup almond milk

1 teaspoon honey

1 teaspoon chia seeds

Instructions:

- Place the blueberries, almonds, and almond milk in a blender.
- Add the honey and chia seeds and blend until smooth.
- Pour into a glass and enjoy!

Nutritional Benefits: This smoothie is packed with antioxidants from the blueberries and healthy fats from the almonds and chia seeds.

Day 1-7 Juicing plan for Boosting Energy and Vitality

Day 1: Beetroot and Carrot Juice

Ingredients:

1 beetroot   2 carrots

1 apple   1 inch ginger

Method:
- Wash the ingredients and blend them all together.
- Strain the juice and drink immediately.

Nutritional Values: Rich in Vitamin C, potassium, iron, and folate.

Day 2: Spinach and Celery Juice

Ingredients:

2 cups spinach   3 celery stalks
1 apple   1/2 lemon (juiced).

Method:

- Wash the ingredients and blend them all together.
- Strain the juice and drink immediately.

Nutritional Values: Rich in Vitamin A, Vitamin C, iron, and magnesium.

Day 3: Pineapple and Ginger Juice

Ingredients:

1/2 pineapple   1 inch ginger
1/2 lemon (juiced)

Method:

- Wash the ingredients and blend them all together
- Strain the juice and drink immediately.

Nutritional Values: Rich in Vitamin C, bromelain, and gingerols.

Day 4: Orange and Turmeric Juice

Ingredients:

3 oranges   1 inch turmeric
1/2 lemon (juiced).

Method:
- Wash the ingredients and blend them all together.
- Strain the juice and drink immediately.

Nutritional Values: Rich in Vitamin C, anti-inflammatory compounds, and antioxidants.

Day 5 Kale and Apple Juice

Ingredients:

2 cups kale   2 apples
1 inch ginger   1/2 lemon (juiced).

Method:
- Wash the ingredients and blend them all together.
- Strain the juice and drink immediately.

Nutritional Values: Rich in Vitamin K, Vitamin C, fiber, and antioxidants.

Day 6: Watermelon and Mint Juice

Ingredients:

1/2 watermelon   1/4 cup mint leaves
1/2 lemon (juiced)

Method:
- Wash the ingredients and blend them all together.

- Strain the juice and drink immediately.

Nutritional Values: Rich in lycopene, potassium, and Vitamin C.

Day 7: Carrot and Ginger Juice

Ingredients:

4 carrots   1 inch ginger
1/2 lemon (juiced)

Method:
- Wash the ingredients and blend them all together.
- Strain the juice and drink immediately.

Nutritional Values: Rich in Vitamin A, Vitamin C, and anti-inflammatory compounds.

These juices should be consumed as a part of a healthy and balanced diet, and not as a replacement for meals.

Day 8-14 Smoothie plan for Improving Digestion and Elimination

Day 8: Apple Pear Ginger Smoothie

Ingredients:

1 apple 1 pear 1-inch knob of ginger

2 cups of almond milk 2 tablespoons of flax seeds

1 teaspoon of honey (optional)

Preparation:

- Peel the ginger, core the apple and pear, and cut them into cubes
- Place all the ingredients in a blender and blend until smooth

- Serve chilled

Nutritional Benefits:

- Rich in antioxidants and anti-inflammatory compounds
- Contains dietary fiber to improve digestion and elimination
- Contains essential vitamins and minerals for overall health

Day 9: Banana Avocado Smoothie

Ingredients:

1 banana / 1 avocado
1 cup of almond milk / 1 tablespoon of chia seeds
1 teaspoon of honey (optional)

Preparation:

- Peel and cut the banana into cubes

- Peel and remove the pit from the avocado, and cut it into cubes
- Place all the ingredients in a blender and blend until smooth
- Serve chilled

Nutritional Benefits:

- Contains dietary fiber to improve digestion and elimination
- Rich in monounsaturated fats and antioxidants
- Contains essential vitamins and minerals for overall health

Day 10: Mango Kale Smoothie

Ingredients:

1 mango   2 cups of kale

1 cup of almond milk

1 tablespoon of hemp seeds

1 teaspoon of honey (optional)

Preparation:

- Peel the mango and cut it into cubes
- Place all the ingredients in a blender and blend until smooth
- Serve chilled

Nutritional Benefits:

- Rich in antioxidants and anti-inflammatory compounds
- Contains dietary fiber to improve digestion and elimination
- Contains essential vitamins and minerals for overall health

Day 11: Strawberry Spinach Smoothie

Ingredients:

1 cup of strawberries   2 cups of spinach

1 cup of almond milk

1 tablespoon of sunflower seeds

1 teaspoon of honey (optional)

Preparation:

- Hull the strawberries and cut them into halves
- Place all the ingredients in a blender and blend until smooth
- Serve chilled

Nutritional Benefits:

- Rich in antioxidants and anti-inflammatory compounds
- Contains dietary fiber to improve digestion and elimination

- Contains essential vitamins and minerals for overall health

Day 12: Carrot Orange Smoothie

Ingredients:

2 carrots   2 oranges

1 cup of almond milk

1 tablespoon of pumpkin seeds

1 teaspoon of honey (optional)

Preparation:

- Peel the carrots and oranges and cut them into cubes
- Place all the ingredients in a blender and blend until smooth
- Serve chilled

Nutritional Benefits:

- Rich in antioxidants and anti-inflammatory compounds
- Contains dietary fiber to improve digestion and elimination
- Contains essential vitamins and minerals for overall health

Day 13: Pineapple Blueberry Smoothie

Ingredients:

1 cup of pineapple   1 cup of blueberries

1 cup of almond milk

1 tablespoon of sesame seeds

1 teaspoon of honey (optional)

Preparation:

- Core the pineapple and cut it into cubes
- Place all the ingredients in a blender and blend until smooth
- Serve chilled

Nutritional Benefits:

- Rich in antioxidants and anti-inflammatory compounds
- Contains dietary fiber to improve digestion and elimination
- Contains essential vitamins and minerals for overall health

Day 14: Cucumber Melon Smoothie

Ingredients:

½ cucumber   ½ melon

1 cup of almond milk

1 tablespoon of quinoa

1 teaspoon of honey (optional)

Preparation:

- Peel the cucumber and cut it into cubes
- Peel, deseed and cut the melon into cubes
- Place all the ingredients in a blender and blend until smooth
- Serve chilled

Nutritional Benefits:

- Rich in antioxidants and anti-inflammatory compounds
- Contains dietary fiber to improve digestion and elimination
- Contains essential vitamins and minerals for overall health

Day 8-14 Juicing plan for Digestion and Elimination

Day 8: Apple Beet Carrot Juice

Ingredients:

3 apples   2 beets   2 carrots

Preparation:

- Core the apples, peel the beets and carrots, and cut them into cubes
- Place all the ingredients in a juicer and extract the juice
- Serve chilled

Nutritional Benefits:

- Rich in antioxidants and anti-inflammatory compounds
- Contains dietary fiber to improve digestion and elimination
- Contains essential vitamins and minerals for overall health

Day 9. Carrot Orange Juice

Ingredients:

4 carrots   2 oranges

Preparation:

- Peel the carrots and oranges and cut them into cubes
- Place all the ingredients in a juicer and extract the juice
- Serve chilled

Nutritional Benefits:

- Rich in antioxidants and anti-inflammatory compounds
- Contains dietary fiber to improve digestion and elimination
- Contains essential vitamins and minerals for overall health

Day 10. Cucumber Celery Ginger Juice

Ingredients:

1 cucumber   2 stalks of celery
1-inch knob of ginger

Preparation:

- Peel the cucumber, celery and ginger, and cut them into cubes
- Place all the ingredients in a juicer and extract the juice
- Serve chilled

Day 11. Kale Spinach Lemon Juice

Ingredients:

2 cups of kale   2 cups of spinach

1 lemon

Preparation:

- Peel the lemon and cut it into wedges
- Place all the ingredients in a juicer and extract the juice
- Serve chilled

Day 12. Pear Apple Ginger Juice

Ingredients:

2 pears   2 apples   1-inch knob of ginger

Preparation:

- Core the pears and apples, peel the ginger, and cut them into cubes

- Place all the ingredients in a juicer and extract the juice
- Serve chilled

Day 13. Beet Carrot Lemon Juice

Ingredients:

2 beets   2 carrots   1 lemon

Preparation:

- Peel the beets and carrots, and cut them into cubes
- Peel the lemon and cut it into wedges
- Place all the ingredients in a juicer and extract the juice
- Serve chilled

Nutritional Benefits:

- Rich in antioxidants and anti-inflammatory compounds
- Contains dietary fiber to improve digestion and elimination
- Contains essential vitamins and minerals for overall health

Day 14. Grapefruit Pineapple Juice

Ingredients:

1 grapefruit   1 cup of pineapple

Preparation:

- Peel the grapefruit and cut it into wedges
- Core the pineapple and cut it into cubes
- Place all the ingredients in a juicer and extract the juice

- Serve chilled

Nutritional Benefits:

- Rich in antioxidants and anti-inflammatory compounds
- Contains dietary fiber to improve digestion and elimination
- Contains essential vitamins and minerals for overall health

Day 15-21 Smoothie plan for Reducing Inflammation and Promoting Joint Health

Day 15: Blueberry, Spinach, and Banana Smoothie:

Ingredients:

- 1 cup of fresh blueberries
- 1 cup of fresh spinach
- 1 banana
- 1 cup of almond milk.

Preparation Method:

Blend all ingredients together until smooth.

Nutritional Benefits: This smoothie is rich in antioxidants and anti-inflammatory compounds, which can help reduce inflammation and support joint health. It is also high in potassium and magnesium, which can help reduce muscle cramps.

Day 16. Avocado, Ginger, and Turmeric Smoothie:

Ingredients:

½ avocado   1 inch piece of ginger

½ teaspoon of turmeric powder

1 cup of almond milk.

Preparation Method:

Blend all ingredients together until smooth.

Nutritional Benefits: This smoothie is rich in healthy fats and antioxidants, which can help reduce inflammation and support joint health. Ginger and turmeric are both anti-inflammatory and can help reduce joint pain.

Day 17. Apple, Kale, and Flaxseed Smoothie:

Ingredients:

1 apple   1 cup of kale

1 tablespoon of ground flaxseed

1 cup of almond milk.

Preparation Method:

Blend all ingredients together until smooth.

Nutritional Benefits: This smoothie is high in **omega-3 fatty acids,** which can help reduce inflammation and support joint health. The kale is also a great source of antioxidants and vitamins, which can help support overall health.

Day 18. Carrot, Celery, and Almond Butter Smoothie:

Ingredients:

2 carrots   2 celery stalks

2 tablespoons of almond butter

1 cup of almond milk.

Preparation Method: Blend all ingredients together until smooth.

Nutritional Benefits: This smoothie is high in **magnesium and potassium**, which can help reduce muscle cramps and support joint health. Almond butter is also a great source of healthy fats, which can help reduce inflammation.

Day 19: Pineapple, Spinach, and Coconut Oil Smoothie:

Ingredients:

1 cup of pineapple   1 cup of spinach

1 tablespoon of coconut oil

1 cup of almond milk.

Preparation Method: Blend all ingredients together until smooth.

Nutritional Benefits: This smoothie is high in **Vitamin C and antioxidants,** which can help reduce inflammation and support joint health. Coconut oil is also a great source of healthy fats, which can help reduce inflammation.

Day 20. Watermelon, Cucumber, and Hemp Seeds Smoothie:

Ingredients:

1 cup of watermelon   ½ cucumber

1 tablespoon of hemp seeds

1 cup of almond milk.

Preparation Method: Blend all ingredients together until smooth.

Nutritional Benefits: This smoothie is high in **Vitamin A and antioxidants,** which can help reduce inflammation and support joint health. The hemp seeds are also a great source of **omega-3 fatty acids,** which can help reduce inflammation.

Day 21: Banana, Oats, and Chia Seeds Smoothie:

Ingredients:

- 1 banana   ½ cup of oats
- 1 tablespoon of chia seeds
- 1 cup of almond milk.

Preparation Method: Blend all ingredients together until smooth.

Nutritional Benefits: This smoothie is **high in fiber**, which can help support healthy digestion and support joint health. The chia seeds are also a great source of omega-3 fatty acids, which can help reduce inflammation.

Day 15-21 Juicing plan for Reducing Inflammation and Promoting Joint Health

Day 15: Carrot, Apple, and Ginger Juice:

Ingredients:

4 carrots   2 apples   1 inch piece of ginger.

Preparation Method: Juice all ingredients together and serve.

Nutritional Benefits: This juice is high in **Vitamin A and antioxidants**, which can help reduce inflammation and support joint health. Ginger is also anti-inflammatory and can help reduce joint pain.

Day 16. Beet, Celery, and Lemon Juice:

Ingredients:

1 beet   2 celery stalks   ½ lemon.

Preparation Method: Juice all ingredients together and serve.

Nutritional Benefits: This juice is high in **antioxidants and anti-inflammatory compounds,** which can help reduce inflammation and support joint health. The lemon is also high in **Vitamin C,** which can help support overall health.

Day 17. Cucumber, Kale, and Turmeric Juice:

Ingredients:

½ cucumber   1 cup of kale

½ teaspoon of turmeric powder.

Preparation Method: Juice all ingredients together and serve.

Nutritional Benefits: This juice is high in **Vitamin A and antioxidants,** which can help reduce inflammation and support joint health. Turmeric is also anti-inflammatory and can help reduce joint pain.

Day 18. Spinach, Parsley, and Lime Juice:

Ingredients:

1 cup of spinach   ½ cup of parsley

½ lime.

Preparation Method: Juice all ingredients together and serve.

Nutritional Benefits: This juice is rich in antioxidants and anti-inflammatory compounds, which can help reduce inflammation and support joint health. The **lime** is also high in **Vitamin C**, which can help support overall health.

Day 19: Watermelon, Broccoli, and Chia Seeds Juice:

Ingredients:

1 cup of watermelon   ½ cup of broccoli

1 tablespoon of chia seeds.

Preparation Method: Juice all ingredients together and serve.

Nutritional Benefits: This juice is high in Vitamin A and antioxidants, which can help reduce inflammation and support joint health. The chia seeds are also a great source of omega-3 fatty acids, which can help reduce inflammation.

Day 20. Apple, Carrot, and Flaxseed Juice:

Ingredients:

2 apples   4 carrots

1 tablespoon of ground flaxseed.

Preparation Method: Juice all ingredients together and serve.

Nutritional Benefits: This juice is high in fiber, which can help support healthy digestion and support joint health. The flaxseed is also a great source of omega-3 fatty acids, which can help reduce inflammation.

Day 21. Pineapple, Cucumber, and Coconut Oil Juice:

Ingredients:

1 cup of pineapple   ½ cucumber

1 tablespoon of coconut oil.

Preparation Method: Juice all ingredients together and serve. Nutritional Benefits: This juice is high in Vitamin C and antioxidants, which can help reduce inflammation and support joint health. The coconut oil is also a great source of healthy fats, which can help reduce inflammation.

Day 22-28 Smoothie plan for Supporting Brain Health and Memory

Day 22 Blueberry Coconut Smoothie

Ingredients:

1 cup of blueberries

1/2 cup of coconut milk   1/2 banana

1 tablespoon of honey

1 tablespoon of chia seeds

Preparation:

Put the ingredients in a blender and blend until you get the texture you want.

Nutritional Benefits:

- Blueberries are packed full of antioxidants, which help protect the brain from oxidative damage.
- Coconut milk is rich in healthy fats and minerals, which help support brain health.
- Bananas are a good source of potassium and magnesium, which help reduce stress and improve memory.

- Honey is a natural sweetener, which provides a boost of energy to the body.
- Chia seeds are a good source of omega-3 fatty acids, which help support brain health and memory.

Day 23: Mango Avocado Smoothie

Ingredients:

1 cup of mango   1/2 avocado

1/2 cup of almond milk

1 tablespoon of honey

1 teaspoon of spirulina

Preparation:

- Place all ingredients into a blender and blend until the desired consistency is achieved.

Nutritional Benefits:

- Mangoes are rich in vitamins, minerals, and antioxidants, which help protect the brain from oxidative damage.
- Avocado is a good source of healthy fats and nutrients, which help support brain health.
- Almond milk is high in calcium and vitamin E, which help improve memory and cognitive function.
- Honey is a natural sweetener, which provides a boost of energy to the body.
- Spirulina is a high source of antioxidants, which help protect the brain and promote memory.

Day 24: Coconut Strawberry Smoothie

Ingredients:

1 cup of strawberries

1/2 cup of coconut milk

1 tablespoon of honey

1 tablespoon of flaxseed oil

1 teaspoon of maca powder

Preparation:

- Put the ingredients in a blender and blend until you get the texture you want.

Nutritional Benefits:

- Strawberries are a good source of vitamin C, which helps protect the brain from oxidative damage.

- Coconut milk is rich in healthy fats and minerals, which help support brain health.

- Honey is a natural sweetener, which provides a boost of energy to the body.

- Flaxseed oil is a good source of omega-3 fatty acids, which help support brain health and memory.

- Maca powder is a high source of antioxidants, which help protect the brain and promote memory.

Day 25: Pineapple Coconut Smoothie

Ingredients:

- 1 cup of pineapple

- 1/2 cup of coconut milk
- 1 tablespoon of honey
- 1 tablespoon of chia seeds
- 1 teaspoon of turmeric powder

Preparation:

- Put the ingredients in a blender and blend until you get the texture you want.

Nutritional Benefits:

- Pineapple is rich in vitamins, minerals, and antioxidants, which help protect the brain from oxidative damage.
- Coconut milk is rich in healthy fats and minerals, which help support brain health.

- Honey is a natural sweetener, which provides a boost of energy to the body.
- Chia seeds are a good source of omega-3 fatty acids, which help support brain health and memory.
- Turmeric powder is a high source of antioxidants, which help protect the brain and promote memory.

Day 26: Banana Avocado Smoothie

Ingredients:

- 1 banana   1/2 avocado
- 1/2 cup of almond milk
- 1 tablespoon of honey
- 1 teaspoon of spirulina

Preparation:

Put the ingredients in a blender and blend until you get the texture you want.

Nutritional Benefits:

- Bananas are a good source of potassium and magnesium, which help reduce stress and improve memory.
- Avocado is a good source of healthy fats and nutrients, which help support brain health.
- Almond milk is high in calcium and vitamin E, which help improve memory and cognitive function.
- Honey is a natural sweetener, which provides a boost of energy to the body.
- Spirulina is a high source of antioxidants, which help protect the brain and promote memory.

Day 27 Acai Berry Smoothie

Ingredients:

- 1 cup of acai berry
- 1/2 cup of almond milk
- 1 tablespoon of honey
- 1 tablespoon of flaxseed oil
- 1 teaspoon of maca powder

Preparation:

Put the ingredients in a blender and blend until you get the texture you want.

Nutritional Benefits:

- Acai berries are a good source of antioxidants, which help protect the brain from oxidative damage.
- Almond milk is high in calcium and vitamin E, which help improve memory and cognitive function.

- Honey is a natural sweetener, which provides a boost of energy to the body.
- Flaxseed oil is a good source of omega-3 fatty acids, which help support brain health and memory.
- Maca powder is a high source of antioxidants, which help protect the brain and promote memory.

Day 28: Avocado Banana Smoothie

Ingredients:

- 1/2 avocado
- 1 banana
- 1/2 cup of coconut milk
- 1 tablespoon of honey
- 1 teaspoon of turmeric powder

Preparation:

Put the ingredients in a blender and blend until you get the texture you want.

Nutritional Benefits:

- Avocado is a good source of healthy fats and nutrients, which help support brain health.
- Bananas are a good source of potassium and magnesium, which help reduce stress and improve memory.
- Coconut milk is rich in healthy fats and minerals, which help support brain health.
- Honey is a natural sweetener, which provides a boost of energy to the body.
- Turmeric powder is a high source of antioxidants, which help protect the brain and promote memory.

Day 22-28 Juicing plan for Supporting Brain Health and Memory

Day 22: Carrot Ginger Juice

Ingredients:

2 carrots

1/2 inch ginger

1/2 cup pineapple

1/2 cup orange juice

Preparation:

- Wash and peel the carrots and ginger.
- Place all the ingredients in a juicer and extract the juice

Nutritional Benefits:

- Carrots are a good source of beta-carotene, which helps protect the brain from oxidative damage.
- Ginger is a natural anti-inflammatory, which helps reduce inflammation in the brain.
- Pineapple is a good source of antioxidants, which help protect the brain and promote memory.
- Orange juice is high in vitamin C, which helps improve memory and cognitive function.

Day 23: Beetroot Apple Juice

Ingredients:

- 1 beetroot   1 apple
- 1/2 cup of carrot juice
- 1/2 cup of orange juice

Preparation:

- Wash and peel the beetroot and apple.
- Place all the ingredients in a juicer and extract the juice

Nutritional Benefits:

- Beetroot is a good source of antioxidants, which help protect the brain from oxidative damage.
- Apples are packed with vitamins, minerals, and antioxidants, which help protect the brain and promote memory.
- Carrot juice is high in beta-carotene, which helps improve memory and cognitive function.

- Orange juice is high in vitamin C, which helps improve memory and cognitive function.

Day 24: Spinach Celery Juice

Ingredients:

- 1 cup spinach
- 1 celery stalk
- 1/2 cup of pineapple juice
- 1/2 cup of apple juice

Preparation:

- Wash and chop the spinach and celery.
- Place all the ingredients in a juicer and extract the juice

Nutritional Benefits:

- Spinach is a good source of folate, which helps protect the brain from oxidative damage.
- Celery is a natural anti-inflammatory, which helps reduce inflammation in the brain.
- Pineapple juice is packed with antioxidants, which help protect the brain and promote memory.
- Apple juice is high in vitamin C, which helps improve memory and cognitive function.

Day 25: Kale Apple Juice

Ingredients:

- 1 cup of kale   1 apple
- 1/2 cup of carrot juice
- 1/2 cup of orange juice

Preparation:

- Wash and chop the kale and apple.
- Place all the ingredients in a juicer and extract the juice

Nutritional Benefits:

- Kale is a good source of vitamin K, which helps protect the brain from oxidative damage.
- Apples are packed with vitamins, minerals, and antioxidants, which help protect the brain and promote memory.
- Carrot juice is high in beta-carotene, which helps improve memory and cognitive function.

- Orange juice is high in vitamin C, which helps improve memory and cognitive function.

Day 26: Cucumber Lemon Juice

Ingredients:

- 1 cucumber   1 lemon
- 1/2 cup of pineapple juice
- 1/2 cup of apple juice

Preparation:

- Wash and peel the cucumber and lemon.
- Place all the ingredients in a juicer and extract the juice

Nutritional Benefits:

- Cucumbers are a good source of antioxidants, which help protect the brain from oxidative damage.
- Lemons are high in vitamin C, which helps improve memory and cognitive function.
- Pineapple juice is packed with antioxidants, which help protect the brain and promote memory.
- Apple juice is high in vitamin C, which helps improve memory and cognitive function.

Day 27: Carrot Turmeric Juice

Ingredients:

- 2 carrots
- 1 teaspoon of turmeric powder
- 1/2 cup of pineapple juice

- 1/2 cup of orange juice

Preparation:

- Wash and peel the carrots.
- Place all the ingredients in a juicer and extract the juice

Nutritional Benefits:

- Carrots are a good source of beta-carotene, which helps protect the brain from oxidative damage.
- Turmeric powder is a high source of antioxidants, which help protect the brain and promote memory.
- Pineapple juice is packed with antioxidants, which help protect the brain and promote memory.

- Orange juice is high in vitamin C, which helps improve memory and cognitive function.

Day 28: Broccoli Apple Juice

Ingredients:

- 1 cup of broccoli
- 1 apple
- 1/2 cup of carrot juice
- 1/2 cup of orange juice

Preparation:

- Wash and chop the broccoli and apple.
- Place all the ingredients in a juicer and extract the juice

Nutritional Benefits:

- Broccoli is a good source of folate, which helps protect the brain from oxidative damage.

- Apples are packed with vitamins, minerals, and antioxidants, which help protect the brain and promote memory.

- Carrot juice is high in beta-carotene, which helps improve memory and cognitive function.

- Orange juice is high in vitamin C, which helps improve memory and cognitive function.

CHAPTER THREE

THE 62-DAY JUICING AND SMOOTHIES PLAN (DAY 29-62)

Day 29-35 Smoothie for Boosting Immunity and Fighting Infections

Day 29: Immune-Boosting Green Smoothie

Ingredients:

1 cup spinach

1 cup kale

½ cup pineapple

½ cup frozen mango

1 banana

1 tablespoon chia seeds

1 tablespoon hemp seeds

1 cup almond milk

Preparation Method:

- Place spinach, kale, pineapple, mango, banana, chia seeds, hemp seeds, and almond milk in a blender.
- Blend until smooth.
- Pour into a glass and enjoy!

Nutritional Benefits: This smoothie is packed with vitamins, minerals, and antioxidants that help to boost the immune system and fight off infections. It is high in vitamin A, which helps to promote healthy vision and skin, and vitamin C, which helps to reduce inflammation and fight off infections. It is also a great source of fiber, which helps to keep the digestive system healthy and keep the body regular.

Day 30: Turmeric Ginger Smoothie

Ingredients:

- 1 cup frozen mango
- ½ cup fresh pineapple
- 1 teaspoon ground turmeric
- 1 teaspoon ground ginger
- 1 banana
- 1 tablespoon chia seeds
- 1 cup almond milk

Preparation Method:

- Place mango, pineapple, turmeric, ginger, banana, chia seeds, and almond milk in a blender.
- Blend until smooth.
- Pour into a glass and enjoy!

Nutritional Benefits: This smoothie is an excellent source of vitamins and minerals that help to boost the immune system and fight off infections. The combination of turmeric and ginger helps to reduce inflammation and boost the body's natural defenses. It is also high in vitamin C, which helps to reduce inflammation and increase the body's natural immunity.

Day 31: Immune-Boosting Berry Smoothie

Ingredients:

- 1 cup frozen blueberries
- ½ cup frozen raspberries
- ½ cup frozen strawberries
- 1 banana
- 1 tablespoon chia seeds

- 1 cup almond milk

Preparation Method:

- Place blueberries, raspberries, strawberries, banana, chia seeds, and almond milk in a blender.
- Blend until smooth.
- Pour into a glass and enjoy!

Nutritional Benefits: This smoothie is packed with antioxidants that help to boost the immune system and fight off infections. It is high in vitamin C, which helps to reduce inflammation and boost the body's natural defenses. It is also a great source of fiber, which helps to keep the digestive system healthy and keep the body regular.

Day 32: Vitamin C Smoothie

Ingredients:

- 1 cup frozen pineapple
- ½ cup frozen mango
- ½ cup frozen strawberries
- 1 banana
- 1 tablespoon chia seeds
- 1 cup orange juice

Preparation Method:

- Place pineapple, mango, strawberries, banana, chia seeds, and orange juice in a blender.
- Blend until smooth.
- Pour into a glass and enjoy!

Nutritional Benefits: This smoothie is an excellent source of vitamin C, which helps to reduce inflammation and fight off infections. It is also a great source of fiber, which helps to keep the digestive system healthy and keep the body regular.

Day 33: Citrus Smoothie

Ingredients:

- 1 cup frozen pineapple
- ½ cup frozen mango
- ½ cup frozen strawberries
- 1 orange, peeled and quartered
- 1 banana
- 1 tablespoon chia seeds
- 1 cup orange juice

Preparation Method:

- Place pineapple, mango, strawberries, orange, banana, chia seeds, and orange juice in a blender.
- Blend until smooth.

- Pour into a glass and enjoy!

Nutritional Benefits: This smoothie is an excellent source of vitamin C, which helps to reduce inflammation and fight off infections. It is also a great source of fiber, which helps to keep the digestive system healthy and keep the body regular. The orange adds a boost of antioxidants, which helps to fight off free radicals and protect the body from damage.

Day 34: Immune-Boosting Beet Smoothie

Ingredients:

- 1 cup frozen beets
- ½ cup frozen strawberries
- ½ cup frozen pineapple
- 1 banana

- 1 tablespoon chia seeds
- 1 cup almond milk

Preparation Method:

- Place beets, strawberries, pineapple, banana, chia seeds, and almond milk in a blender.
- Blend until smooth.
- Pour into a glass and enjoy!

Nutritional Benefits: This smoothie is packed with vitamins, minerals, and antioxidants that help to boost the immune system and fight off infections. It is high in vitamin C, which helps to reduce inflammation and fight off infections. The beets are an excellent source of folate, which helps to promote healthy cell growth and development.

Day 35: Immune-Boosting Carrot Smoothie

Ingredients:

- 1 cup frozen carrots
- ½ cup frozen mango
- ½ cup frozen pineapple
- 1 banana
- 1 tablespoon chia seeds
- 1 cup almond milk

Preparation Method:

- Place carrots, mango, pineapple, banana, chia seeds, and almond milk in a blender.
- Blend until smooth.
- Pour into a glass and enjoy!

Nutritional Benefits: This smoothie is an excellent source of vitamins and minerals that help to boost the immune system and fight off infections. It is high in vitamin A, which helps to promote healthy vision and skin, and vitamin C, which helps to reduce inflammation and fight off infections. The carrots are also a great source of beta-carotene, which helps to protect the body from damage caused by free radicals.

Day 29-35 Juicing for Boosting Immunity and Fighting Infections

Day 29: Immune-Boosting Green Juice

Ingredients:

1 cup kale	1 cup spinach
½ cucumber	1 apple
1 lemon, peeled	1 inch ginger root

Preparation Method:

- Place kale, spinach, cucumber, apple, lemon, and ginger root in a juicer.
- Place all the ingredients in a juicer and extract the juice
- Pour into a glass and enjoy!

Nutritional Benefits: This juice is packed with vitamins, minerals, and antioxidants that help to boost the immune system and fight off infections. It is high in vitamin C, which helps to reduce inflammation and fight off infections. The lemon adds a boost of vitamin C, while the ginger helps to reduce inflammation and promote healthy digestion.

Day 30: Citrus Juice

Ingredients:

- 1 orange, peeled
- 1 grapefruit, peeled
- 1 lemon, peeled
- 1 inch ginger root

Preparation Method:

- Place orange, grapefruit, lemon, and ginger root in a juicer.
- Place all the ingredients in a juicer and extract the juice
- Pour into a glass and enjoy!

Nutritional Benefits: This juice is packed with vitamins, minerals, and antioxidants that help to boost the immune system and fight off infections. The combination of citrus fruits provides a boost of vitamin C, while the ginger helps to reduce inflammation and promote healthy digestion.

Day 31: Immune-Boosting Beet Juice

Ingredients:

2 beets	1 apple
1 lemon, peeled	1 inch ginger root

Preparation Method:

- Place beets, apple, lemon, and ginger root in a juicer.
- Place all the ingredients in a juicer and extract the juice
- Pour into a glass and enjoy!

Nutritional Benefits: This juice is packed with vitamins, minerals, and antioxidants that help to boost the immune system and fight off infections. The beets are an excellent source of folate, which helps to promote healthy cell growth and development. The combination of citrus fruits provides a boost of vitamin C, while the ginger helps to reduce inflammation and promote healthy digestion.

Day 32: Immune-Boosting Carrot Juice

Ingredients:

2 carrots   1 apple

1 lemon, peeled   1 inch ginger root

Preparation Method:

- Place carrots, apple, lemon, and ginger root in a juicer.
- Place all the ingredients in a juicer and extract the juice
- Pour into a glass and enjoy!

Nutritional Benefits: This juice is packed with vitamins, minerals, and antioxidants that help to boost the immune system and fight off infections. The carrots are an excellent source of beta-carotene, which helps to protect the body from damage caused by free radicals. The combination of citrus fruits provides a boost of vitamin C, while the ginger helps to reduce inflammation and promote healthy digestion.

Day 33: Immune-Boosting Ginger Juice

Ingredients:

1 apple   1 lemon, peeled
1 inch ginger root   1 cup water

Preparation Method:

- Place apple, lemon, ginger root, and water in a juicer.
- Place all the ingredients in a juicer and extract the juice
- Pour into a glass and enjoy!

Nutritional Benefits: This juice is an excellent source of vitamins and minerals that help to boost the immune system and fight off infections. Ginger helps to reduce inflammation and promote healthy digestion. It is also high in vitamin C, which helps to reduce inflammation and increase the body's natural immunity.

Day 34: Immune-Boosting Apple Juice

Ingredients:

3 apples   1 lemon, peeled

1 inch ginger root

Preparation Method:

- Place apples, lemon, and ginger root in a juicer.
- Place all the ingredients in a juicer and extract the juice
- Pour into a glass and enjoy!

Nutritional Benefits: This juice is packed with vitamins, minerals, and antioxidants that help to boost the immune system and fight off infections. The apples are an excellent source of fiber, which helps to keep the digestive system healthy and keep the body regular. The combination of citrus fruits provides a boost of vitamin C, while the ginger helps to reduce inflammation and promote healthy digestion.

Day 35: Immune-Boosting Turmeric Juice

Ingredients:

1 apple   1 lemon, peeled

1 inch ginger root

1 teaspoon ground turmeric

Preparation Method:

- Place apple, lemon, ginger root, and turmeric in a juicer.

- Place all the ingredients in a juicer and extract the juice

- Pour into a glass and enjoy!

Nutritional Benefits: This juice is an excellent source of vitamins and minerals that help to boost the immune system and fight off infections. The combination of ginger and turmeric helps to reduce inflammation and boost the body's natural defenses. It is also high in vitamin C, which helps to reduce inflammation and increase the body's natural immunity.

Day 36-42 Smoothie to Promote Heart Health and Lowering Cholesterol

Day 36: Strawberry and Banana Smoothie

Ingredients:

- 1 banana
- 1 cup fresh or frozen strawberries
- 1 cup plain Greek yogurt
- 1 teaspoon lemon juice
- ½ cup almond milk
- 2 tablespoons honey

Preparation Method:

- In a blender, combine the banana, strawberries, yogurt, lemon juice, almond milk, and honey.

- Blend until smooth.
- Pour into glasses and enjoy!

Nutritional Benefits: This delicious smoothie is high in fiber and Vitamin C, which helps to promote heart health and lower cholesterol. It is also packed with protein from the Greek yogurt, and healthy fats from the almond milk, which helps to keep you full and energized.

Day 37: Blueberry and Oatmeal Smoothie

Ingredients:

- 1 cup frozen blueberries
- ½ cup rolled oats
- 1 cup low-fat milk
- 1 tablespoon honey
- ½ teaspoon vanilla extract

Preparation Method:

- Put all the ingredients into a blender and mix until it becomes creamy.
- Pour into glasses and enjoy!

Nutritional Benefits: This smoothie is a great way to get your daily dose of antioxidants and fiber, which helps to promote heart health and lower cholesterol. Oatmeal is also a great source of whole grains and helps to keep you full longer.

Day 38: Peach and Spinach Smoothie

Ingredients:

- 1 cup frozen peaches
- 1 cup baby spinach
- ½ cup plain Greek yogurt
- ½ cup almond milk

- 1 teaspoon honey

Preparation Method:

- Put all the ingredients into a blender and mix until it becomes creamy.
- Pour into glasses and enjoy!

Nutritional Benefits: This smoothie is full of vitamins and minerals, including Vitamin A and Iron. It is also high in fiber and protein, which helps to promote heart health and lower cholesterol. The almond milk adds healthy fats to help keep you full and energized.

Day 39: Avocado and Banana Smoothie

Ingredients:

1 banana   ½ avocado

1 cup low-fat milk   1 teaspoon honey

½ teaspoon vanilla extract

Preparation Method:

- Put all the ingredients into a blender and mix until it becomes creamy.
- Pour into glasses and enjoy!

Nutritional Benefits: This smoothie is high in healthy fats, which helps to promote heart health and lower cholesterol. It is also packed with fiber and Vitamin B6, which helps to keep you full and energized.

Day 40: Coconut and Mango Smoothie

Ingredients:

1 cup frozen mango   ½ cup coconut milk

1 teaspoon honey   1 teaspoon chia seeds

½ teaspoon vanilla extract

Preparation Method:

- Put all the ingredients into a blender and mix until it becomes creamy.
- Pour into glasses and enjoy!

Nutritional Benefits: This smoothie is high in healthy fats and Vitamin C, which helps to promote heart health and lower cholesterol. The chia seeds are a great source of Omega-3 fatty acids, which helps to reduce inflammation.

Day 41: Pineapple and Green Tea Smoothie

Ingredients:

- 1 cup frozen pineapple

- 1 cup brewed green tea

- 1 teaspoon honey

- ½ teaspoon ground ginger

Preparation Method:

- Put all the ingredients into a blender and mix until it becomes creamy.

- Pour into glasses and enjoy!

Nutritional Benefits: This smoothie is packed with antioxidants and polyphenols, which helps to promote heart health and lower cholesterol. The ginger adds an extra boost of anti-inflammatory benefits, and the honey adds just the right amount of sweetness.

Day 42: Vanilla and Acai Berry Smoothie

Ingredients:

- ½ cup frozen acai berries
- 1 cup almond milk
- 1 teaspoon honey
- ½ teaspoon vanilla extract

Preparation Method:

- Put all the ingredients into a blender and mix until it becomes creamy.
- Pour into glasses and enjoy!

Nutritional Benefits: This smoothie is packed with antioxidants and healthy fats, which helps to promote heart health and lower cholesterol. The acai berries are a great source of fiber and Vitamin C, and the almond milk adds an extra boost of healthy fats.

Day 36-42 Juicing plan to Promote Heart Health and Lowering Cholesterol

Day 36: Beet and Carrot Juice

Ingredients:

1 beet   2 carrots

1 apple   1 lemon

Preparation Method:

- Wash and peel the beet and carrots.
- Cut the beet, carrots and apple into small pieces.
- Place all the ingredients into a juicer and process.
- Enjoy your juice.

Nutritional Benefits: This juice is high in fiber and antioxidants, which helps to promote heart health and lower cholesterol. It is also full of Vitamin A and Vitamin C, which helps to boost the immune system.

Day 37: Kale and Apple Juice

Ingredients:

1 cup kale

1 apple

2 carrots

1 lemon

Preparation Method:

- Wash and peel the apple and carrots.
- Cut the apple, carrots and kale into small pieces.
- Place all the ingredients into a juicer and process.

- Enjoy your juice.

Nutritional Benefits: This juice is packed with fiber, healthy fats, and vitamins, which helps to promote heart health and lower cholesterol. Kale is a great source of Vitamin C, which helps to boost the immune system.

Day 38: Celery and Cucumber Juice

Ingredients:

2 celery stalks   1 cucumber

1 apple   ½ lemon

Preparation Method:

- Wash and peel the apple and cucumber.

- Cut the apple, cucumber and celery into small pieces.
- Place all the ingredients into a juicer and process.
- Enjoy your juice.

Nutritional Benefits: This juice is full of fiber and minerals, which helps to promote heart health and lower cholesterol. The cucumber is a great source of Vitamin K, which helps with blood clotting.

Day 39: Apple and Parsley Juice

Ingredients:

2 apples	½ cup parsley
1 lemon	2 carrots

Preparation Method:

- Peel the apples and carrots, then wash them.
- Cut the apples, carrots and parsley into small pieces.
- Place all the ingredients into a juicer and process.
- Enjoy your juice.

Nutritional Benefits: This juice is high in Vitamin C and antioxidants, which helps to promote heart health and lower cholesterol. The parsley is a great source of Vitamin A and Vitamin K, which helps to boost the immune system.

Day 40: Cucumber and Ginger Juice

Ingredients:

1 cucumber   1 inch fresh ginger

1 apple   ½ lemon

Preparation Method:

- Wash and peel the cucumber and apple.
- Cut the cucumber, apple and ginger into small pieces.
- Place all the ingredients into a juicer and process.
- Enjoy your juice.

Nutritional Benefits: This juice is full of antioxidants and anti-inflammatory benefits, which helps to promote heart health and lower cholesterol. The ginger adds a boost of Vitamin C, which helps to boost the immune system.

Day 41: Spinach and Pear Juice

<h2 style="text-align:center">Ingredients:</h2>

1 cup spinach	1 pear
1 apple	½ lemon

Preparation Method:

- Wash and peel the pear and apple.
- Cut the pear, apple and spinach into small pieces.
- Place all the ingredients into a juicer and process.
- Enjoy your juice.

Nutritional Benefits: This juice is full of fiber and vitamins, which helps to promote heart health and lower cholesterol. The spinach is a great source of Vitamin A and Vitamin K, which helps to boost the immune system.

Day 42: Pineapple and Orange Juice

Ingredients:

1 cup pineapple   2 oranges

1 lemon

Preparation Method:

- Peel the oranges and lemon.
- Cut the pineapple, oranges and lemon into small pieces.
- Place all the ingredients into a juicer and process.
- Enjoy your juice.

Nutritional Benefits: This juice is high in Vitamin C and antioxidants, which helps to promote heart health and lower cholesterol. The pineapple is a great source of fiber and minerals, which helps to boost the immune system.

Day 43-49 Smoothies to Improves Skin Health and Appearance

Day 43: Green Tea and Kale Smoothie

Ingredients:

- 1 cup of green tea   1 cup of kale
- 1/2 cup of spinach   1 banana
- 1/2 cup of almond milk
- 1 teaspoon of honey
- 1 teaspoon of chia seeds

Instructions:

- Put all the ingredients into the blender and blend until the mixture is creamy.
- Pour into a glass and enjoy!

Nutritional Benefits: This smoothie is packed with antioxidants from the green tea and kale, as well as essential vitamins and minerals from the spinach, banana, and almond milk. The chia seeds are high in omega-3 fatty acids, which are beneficial for skin health and appearance.

Day 44: Avocado and Mango Smoothie

Ingredients:

- 1/2 an avocado   1/2 a mango
- 1/2 cup of Greek yogurt
- 1 cup of almond milk
- 1 teaspoon of chia seeds

- 1 teaspoon of honey

Instructions:

- Put all the ingredients into the blender and blend until the mixture is creamy.
- Pour into a glass and enjoy!

Nutritional Benefits: Avocados are high in healthy fats that are beneficial for skin health and appearance. The mango and Greek yogurt provide essential vitamins and minerals that are beneficial for overall health. The almond milk and chia seeds are also high in omega-3 fatty acids that are great for skin health and appearance.

Day 45: Blueberry, Banana, and Oat Smoothie

Ingredients:

- 1 cup of blueberries   1 banana
- 1/2 cup of rolled oats
- 1 cup of almond milk
- 1 teaspoon of honey
- 1 teaspoon of chia seeds

Instructions:

- Put all the ingredients into the blender and blend until the mixture is creamy.
- Pour into a glass and enjoy!

Nutritional Benefits: Blueberries are packed with antioxidants that are beneficial for skin health and appearance. Bananas provide essential vitamins and minerals that are beneficial for overall health. The rolled oats and almond milk are high in fiber and omega-3 fatty acids, which are beneficial for skin health and appearance.

Day 46: Carrot, Orange, and Flaxseed Smoothie

Ingredients:

- 1 carrot   1 orange
- 1/2 cup of almond milk
- 1 teaspoon of honey
- 1 teaspoon of flaxseed

Instructions:

- Put all the ingredients into the blender and blend until the mixture is creamy.
- Pour into a glass and enjoy!

Nutritional Benefits: Carrots are high in beta-carotene, which is beneficial for skin health and appearance. Oranges provide essential vitamins and minerals that are beneficial for overall health. The almond milk and flaxseed are high in omega-3 fatty acids, which are beneficial for skin health and appearance.

Day 47: Apple, Cinnamon, and Walnut Smoothie

Ingredients:

- 1 apple
- 1 teaspoon of cinnamon
- 1/2 cup of walnuts
- 1 cup of almond milk
- 1 teaspoon of honey
- 1 teaspoon of chia seeds

Instructions:

- Put all the ingredients into the blender and blend until the mixture is creamy.
- Pour into a glass and enjoy!

Nutritional Benefits: Apples are packed with antioxidants that are beneficial for skin health and appearance. Cinnamon is high in anti-inflammatory properties that are beneficial for overall health. Walnuts and almond milk are high in omega-3 fatty acids, which are beneficial for skin health and appearance.

Day 48: Spinach, Pear, and Sunflower Seed Smoothie

Ingredients:

- 1 cup of spinach   1 pear
- 1/2 cup of sunflower seeds
- 1 cup of almond milk
- 1 teaspoon of honey
- 1 teaspoon of chia seeds

Instructions:

- Put all the ingredients into the blender and blend until the mixture is creamy.
- Pour into a glass and enjoy!

Nutritional Benefits: Spinach is high in vitamins and minerals that are beneficial for skin health and appearance. Pears provide essential vitamins and minerals that are beneficial for overall health. Sunflower seeds and almond milk are high in omega-3 fatty acids, which are beneficial for skin health and appearance.

Day 49: Cucumber, Ginger, and Hemp Seed Smoothie

Ingredients:

- 1 cucumber
- 1 teaspoon of ginger
- 1/2 cup of hemp seeds

- 1 cup of almond milk

- 1 teaspoon of honey

- 1 teaspoon of chia seeds

Instructions:

- Put all the ingredients into the blender and blend until the mixture is creamy.

- Pour into a glass and enjoy!

Nutritional Benefits: Cucumbers are high in vitamins and minerals that are beneficial for skin health and appearance. Ginger is also high in anti-inflammatory properties that are beneficial for overall health. Hemp seeds and almond milk are high in omega-3 fatty acids, which are beneficial for skin health and appearance.

Day 43-49 Juicing to Improves Skin Health and Appearance

Day 43: Carrot and Orange Juice

Ingredients:

3 carrots   2 oranges

Instructions:

- Peel and chop oranges and carrots.
- Place in a juicer and extract the juice.
- Pour into a glass and enjoy!

Nutritional Benefits: Carrots are high in beta-carotene, which is beneficial for skin health and appearance. Oranges provide essential vitamins and minerals that are beneficial for overall health.

Day 44: Beet, Apple, and Ginger Juice

Ingredients:

- 1 beet
- 1 apple
- 1 teaspoon of ginger

Instructions:

- Peel and chop the beet, apple, and ginger.
- Place in a juicer and extract the juice.
- Pour into a glass and enjoy!

Nutritional Benefits: Beets are high in antioxidants that are beneficial for skin health and appearance. Apples provide essential vitamins and minerals that are beneficial for overall health. The ginger is high in anti-inflammatory properties that are beneficial for overall health.

Day 45: Kale and Pineapple Juice

Ingredients:

1 cup of kale   1/2 a pineapple

Instructions:

- Chop the kale and pineapple.
- Place in a juicer and extract the juice.
- Pour into a glass and enjoy!

Nutritional Benefits: Kale is packed with antioxidants that are beneficial for skin health and appearance. Pineapple is high in essential vitamins and minerals that are beneficial for overall health.

Day 46: Carrot and Celery Juice

Ingredients:

2 carrots   2 stalks of celery

Instructions:

- Peel and chop the carrots and celery.
- Place in a juicer and extract the juice.
- Pour into a glass and enjoy!

Nutritional Benefits: Carrots are high in beta-carotene, which is beneficial for skin health and appearance. Celery provides essential vitamins and minerals that are beneficial for overall health.

Day 47: Spinach and Pear Juice

Ingredients:

1 cup of spinach   1 pear

Instructions:

- Chop the spinach and pear.
- Place in a juicer and extract the juice.
- Pour into a glass and enjoy!

Nutritional Benefits: Spinach is high in vitamins and minerals that are beneficial for skin health and appearance. Pears provide essential vitamins and minerals that are beneficial for overall health.

Day 48: Cucumber and Parsley Juice

Ingredients:

1 cucumber   1/2 cup of parsley

Instructions:

- Peel and chop the cucumber and parsley.

- Place in a juicer and extract the juice.
- Pour into a glass and enjoy!

Nutritional Benefits: Cucumbers are high in vitamins and minerals that are beneficial for skin health and appearance. Parsley provides essential vitamins and minerals that are beneficial for overall health.

Day 49 - Apple and Cinnamon Juice

Ingredients:

2 apples

1 teaspoon of cinnamon

Instructions:

- Peel and chop the apples.
- Place in a juicer and extract the juice.
- Add the cinnamon and stir.
- Pour into a glass and enjoy!

Nutritional Benefits: Apples are packed with antioxidants that are beneficial for skin health and appearance. Cinnamon is high in anti-inflammatory properties that are beneficial for overall health.

Day 50-56 Smoothies to Supports Bone Health and Preventing Osteoporosis

Day 50: Blueberry Oatmeal Smoothie

Ingredients/Preparation Method:

- Combine 1 cup of frozen blueberries
- 1/2 cup rolled oats
- 1/2 cup almond milk
- 1/2 cup plain Greek yogurt
- 1/2 teaspoon vanilla extract
- 1 teaspoon honey in a blender.

- Blend until smooth.

Nutritional Benefits: This smoothie is packed with antioxidants from the blueberries, fiber and protein from the oats and Greek yogurt, and good fats from the almond milk. The combination of these ingredients helps promote bone health and prevent osteoporosis by providing essential nutrients such as calcium, magnesium, and vitamin D.

Day 51: Banana Spinach Smoothie

Ingredients/Preparation Method:

- In a blender, combine 1 banana
- 1/2 cup baby spinach
- 1/2 cup almond milk
- 1/2 cup plain Greek yogurt
- 1/2 teaspoon vanilla extract

- 1 teaspoon honey
- Blend until smooth.

Nutritional Benefits: This smoothie is packed with vitamin K from the spinach, fiber and protein from the Greek yogurt, and good fats from the almond milk. The combination of these ingredients helps promote bone health and prevent osteoporosis by providing essential nutrients such as calcium, magnesium, and vitamin D.

Day 52: Apple Cinnamon Smoothie

Ingredients/Preparation Method:

- In a blender, combine 1 apple (cored and chopped)
- 1/2 teaspoon ground cinnamon
- 1/2 cup almond milk

- 1/2 cup plain Greek yogurt
- 1/2 teaspoon vanilla extract
- 1 teaspoon honey
- Blend until smooth.

Nutritional Benefits: This smoothie is packed with antioxidants from the apple, fiber and protein from the Greek yogurt, and good fats from the almond milk. The combination of these ingredients helps promote bone health and prevent osteoporosis by providing essential nutrients such as calcium, magnesium, and vitamin D.

Day 53: Coconut Kale Smoothie

Ingredients/Preparation Method:

- In a blender, combine 1/2 cup coconut milk

- 1/2 cup kale (stems removed)
- 1/2 cup plain Greek yogurt
- 1/2 teaspoon vanilla extract and 1 teaspoon honey.
- Blend until smooth.

Nutritional Benefits: This smoothie is packed with vitamin K from the kale, fiber and protein from the Greek yogurt, and good fats from the coconut milk. The combination of these ingredients helps promote bone health and prevent osteoporosis by providing essential nutrients such as calcium, magnesium, and vitamin D.

Day 54: Avocado Pear Smoothie

Ingredients/Preparation Method:

- In a blender, combine 1 avocado (peeled and pitted)
- 1 pear (cored and chopped)
- 1/2 cup almond milk
- 1/2 cup plain Greek yogurt
- 1/2 teaspoon vanilla extract and 1 teaspoon honey.
- Blend until smooth.

Nutritional Benefits: This smoothie is packed with good fats from the avocado, fiber and protein from the Greek yogurt, and good fats from the almond milk. The combination of these ingredients helps promote bone health and prevent osteoporosis by providing essential nutrients such as calcium, magnesium, and vitamin D.

Day 55: Peach Ginger Smoothie

Ingredients/Preparation Method:

- In a blender, combine 2 peaches (pitted and chopped)
- 1/2 teaspoon ground ginger
- 1/2 cup almond milk
- 1/2 cup plain Greek yogurt
- 1/2 teaspoon vanilla extract and 1 teaspoon honey.
- Blend until smooth.

Nutritional Benefits: This smoothie is packed with antioxidants from the peaches, fiber and protein from the Greek yogurt, and good fats from the almond milk. The combination of these ingredients helps promote bone health and prevent osteoporosis by providing essential nutrients such as calcium, magnesium, and vitamin D.

Day 56: Strawberry Banana Smoothie

Ingredients/Preparation Method:

- In a blender, combine 1 cup frozen strawberries
- 1 banana, 1/2 cup almond milk
- 1/2 cup plain Greek yogurt
- 1/2 teaspoon vanilla extract and 1 teaspoon honey
- Blend until smooth.

Nutritional Benefits: This smoothie is packed with antioxidants from the strawberries, fiber and protein from the Greek yogurt, and good fats from the almond milk. The combination of these ingredients helps promote bone health and prevent osteoporosis by providing essential nutrients such as calcium and magnesium.

Day 50-56 Juicing plan to Support Bone Health and Preventing Osteoporosis

Day 50: Carrot Juice

Ingredient

2 carrots

Preparation Method:

- Peel and chop the 2 carrots and add to a juicer and extract the juice

Nutritional Benefits: Carrot juice is packed with beta-carotene, which helps promote bone health and prevent osteoporosis by providing essential nutrients such as calcium, magnesium, and vitamin D.

Day 51: Beet Juice

Preparation Method: Peel and chop 1 beet and add to a juicer and extract the juice

Nutritional Benefits: Beet juice is packed with antioxidants, which helps promote bone health and prevent osteoporosis by providing essential nutrients such as calcium, magnesium, and vitamin D.

Day 52: Celery Juice

Preparation Method: Chop 3 stalks of celery and add to a juicer and extract the juice

Nutritional Benefits: Celery juice is packed with vitamins and minerals, which helps promote bone health and prevent osteoporosis by providing essential nutrients such as calcium, magnesium, and vitamin D.

Day 53: Kale Juice

Preparation Method: Chop 1 cup of kale and add to a juicer and extract the juice

Nutritional Benefits: Kale juice is packed with vitamins and minerals, which helps promote bone health and prevent osteoporosis by providing essential nutrients such as calcium, magnesium, and vitamin D.

Day 54: Spinach Juice

Preparation Method: Chop 1 cup of spinach and add to a juicer and extract the juice.

Nutritional Benefits: Spinach juice is packed with vitamins and minerals, which helps promote bone health and prevent osteoporosis by providing essential nutrients such as calcium, magnesium, and vitamin D.

Day 55: Apple Juice

Preparation Method: Core and chop 2 apples and add to a juicer and extract the juice.

Nutritional Benefits: Apple juice is packed with antioxidants, which helps promote bone health and prevent osteoporosis by providing essential nutrients such as calcium, magnesium, and vitamin D.

Day 56: Orange Juice

Preparation Method: Peel and chop 2 oranges and add to a juicer and extract the juice.

Nutritional Benefits: Orange juice is packed with vitamins and minerals, which helps promote bone health and prevent osteoporosis by providing essential nutrients such as calcium, magnesium, and vitamin D.

Day 57-62 Smoothie for Wrapping Up and Maintaining a Healthy Lifestyle

Day 57: Blueberry Banana Blast

Ingredients:

- 1 banana
- 1/2 cup blueberries
- 1/2 cup almond milk
- 1 tablespoon honey
- 1/2 cup ice cubes

Instructions:

- Put all the ingredients into the blender and blend until the mixture is creamy.
- Serve chilled.

Nutritional Benefits: This smoothie is packed with antioxidants, vitamins, and minerals. The blueberries are a great source of vitamin C and fiber, while the banana provides a boost of potassium and magnesium. The honey is a natural sweetener and the almond milk provides calcium and protein.

Day 58: Peanut Butter and Jelly Smoothie

Ingredients:

- 1 banana
- 1/4 cup natural peanut butter
- 1/2 cup frozen mixed berries
- 1/2 cup almond milk
- 1 tablespoon honey
- 1/2 cup ice cubes

Instructions:

- Put all the ingredients into the blender and blend until the mixture is creamy.
- Serve chilled.

Nutritional Benefits: This smoothie is a great source of protein and healthy fats. The peanut butter provides a boost of healthy fats and the mixed berries provide antioxidants and fiber. The banana adds potassium and magnesium, while the almond milk provides calcium and protein.

Day 59: Kale and Apple Smoothie

Ingredients:

- 1 cup kale leaves
- 1 apple
- 1/2 cup almond milk
- 1 tablespoon honey
- 1/2 cup ice cubes

Instructions:

- Put all the ingredients into the blender and blend until the mixture is creamy.
- Serve chilled.

Nutritional Benefits: This smoothie is packed with vitamins, minerals, and antioxidants. The kale provides a boost of vitamin K, vitamin C, and fiber, while the apple is a great source of vitamin A and fiber. The almond milk provides calcium and protein, and the honey is a natural sweetener.

Day 60: Mango and Coconut Smoothie

Ingredients:

- 1 cup mango
- 1/2 cup coconut milk
- 1/2 cup almond milk
- 1 tablespoon honey
- 1/2 cup ice cubes

Instructions:

Put all the ingredients into the blender and blend until the mixture is creamy.

Serve chilled.

Nutritional Benefits: This smoothie is a great source of vitamin C, potassium, and magnesium. The mango provides a boost of vitamin C and antioxidants, while the coconut milk is a great source of healthy fats. The almond milk provides calcium and protein, and the honey is a natural sweetener.

Day 61: Avocado and Spinach Smoothie

Ingredients:

- 1/2 avocado
- 1 cup spinach

- 1/2 cup almond milk
- 1 tablespoon honey
- 1/2 cup ice cubes

Instructions:

- Put all the ingredients into the blender and blend until the mixture is creamy.
- Serve chilled.

Nutritional Benefits: This smoothie is packed with healthy fats, vitamins, and minerals. The avocado provides a boost of healthy fats, while the spinach provides a boost of vitamin K, vitamin A, and fiber. The almond milk provides calcium and protein, and the honey is a natural sweetener. Smoothie #6: Carrot and Orange Smoothie Ingredients: - 1 carrot - 1 orange - 1/2 cup almond milk - 1 tablespoon honey - 1/2 cup ice cubes   Instructions: 1. Put all the ingredients into the blender and blend until the mixture is creamy.   2. Serve chilled. Nutritional Benefits: This smoothie is a great source of vitamin A and vitamin C. The carrot is a great source of vitamin A, while the orange provides a boost of vitamin C. The almond milk provides calcium and protein, and the honey is a natural sweetener.

Day 62: Banana Oatmeal Smoothie

Ingredients:

- 1 banana
- 1/2 cup rolled oats
- 1/2 cup almond milk
- 1 tablespoon honey
- 1/2 cup ice cubes

Instructions:

- Put all the ingredients into the blender and blend until the mixture is creamy.
- Serve chilled.

Nutritional Benefits: This smoothie is packed with vitamins, minerals, and fiber. The banana provides a boost of potassium and magnesium, while the oats are a great source of fiber. The almond milk provides calcium and protein, and the honey is a natural sweetener.

Day 57-62 juicing plan for Wrapping Up and Maintaining a Healthy Lifestyle

Day 57: Apple, Carrot, and Ginger Juice

Ingredients:

- 2 apples
- 2 carrots
- 1 inch ginger

Instructions:

- Peel and chop the apples, carrots, and ginger.
- Place the ingredients in a juicer and process until smooth.
- Serve chilled.

Nutritional Benefits: This juice is packed with vitamins, minerals, and antioxidants. The apples are a great source of vitamin C and fiber, while the carrots provide a boost of beta-carotene and vitamin A. The ginger adds an anti-inflammatory kick and helps to aid digestion.

Day 58: Cucumber, Celery, and Lemon Juice

Ingredients:

- 1 cucumber
- 2 celery stalks
- 1 lemon

Instructions:

- Peel and chop the cucumber, celery, and lemon.
- Place the ingredients in a juicer and process until smooth.
- Serve chilled.

Nutritional Benefits: This juice is a great source of vitamins, minerals, and antioxidants. The cucumber and celery provide a boost of fiber and vitamin K, while the lemon adds a boost of vitamin C.

Day 59: Beet, Apple, and Carrot Juice

Ingredients:

1 beet　　　　2 apples　　　　2 carrots

Instructions:

- Peel and chop the beet, apples, and carrots.
- Place the ingredients in a juicer and process until smooth.
- Serve chilled.

Nutritional Benefits: This juice is packed with vitamins, minerals, and antioxidants. The beets are a great source of iron, while the apples and carrots provide a boost of vitamin A and vitamin C.

Day 60: Kale, Apple, and Lemon Juice

Ingredients:

- 1 cup kale leaves
- 2 apples
- 1 lemon

Instructions:

- Peel and chop the apples and lemon.
- Place the ingredients in a juicer and process until smooth.
- Serve chilled.

Nutritional Benefits: This juice is packed with vitamins, minerals, and antioxidants. The kale is a great source of vitamin K, while the apples and lemon provide a boost of vitamin C.

Day 61: Spinach, Pear, and Ginger Juice

Ingredients:

- 1 cup spinach
- 2 pears
- 1 inch ginger

Instructions:

- Peel and chop the pears and ginger.
- Place the ingredients in a juicer and process until smooth.
- Serve chilled.

Nutritional Benefits: This juice is a great source of vitamins, minerals, and antioxidants. The spinach provides a boost of vitamin A and vitamin K, while the pears are a great source of fiber. The ginger adds an anti-inflammatory kick and helps to aid digestion.

Day 62: Pineapple, Orange, and Carrot Juice

Ingredients:

- 1 cup pineapple
- 2 oranges
- 2 carrots

Instructions:

- Peel and chop the pineapple, oranges, and carrots.
- Place the ingredients in a juicer and process until smooth.
- Serve chilled.

Nutritional Benefits: This juice is packed with vitamins, minerals, and antioxidants.

The pineapple is a great source of vitamin C, while the oranges and carrots provide a boost of vitamin A.

Day 63: Tomato, Celery, and Lemon Juice

Ingredients:

- 3 tomatoes
- 2 celery stalks
- 1 lemon

Instructions:

- Peel and chop the tomatoes, celery, and lemon.
- Place the ingredients in a juicer and process until smooth.
- Serve chilled.

Nutritional Benefits: This juice is a great source of vitamins, minerals, and antioxidants. The tomatoes are a great source of lycopene, while the celery and lemon provide a boost of vitamin K and vitamin C.

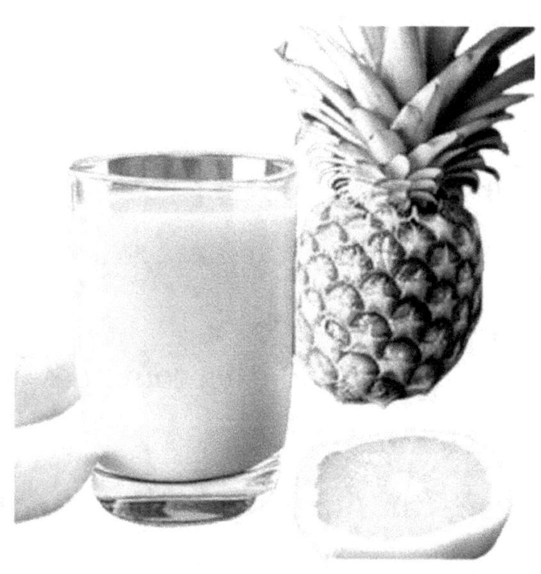

CHAPTER FOUR

MAKING TIME FOR JUICING AND SMOOTHIE MAKING

For seniors over 60, making time for juicing and smoothie making is an important part of staying healthy and active. Juicing and smoothies can provide seniors with many essential vitamins, minerals, and other nutrients that are beneficial for overall health and vitality. By incorporating juicing and smoothie making into their daily routine, seniors can easily increase their intake of these important nutrients, which can help to improve their physical and mental wellbeing. Juicing and smoothie making can also help seniors to maintain a healthy weight.

Juicing and smoothies are a great way to get in extra servings of fruits and vegetables without the calories and fat that can come with more traditional meals. Juicing and smoothies can also be a great way to add additional protein and fiber to one's diet.

The added fiber can help to keep seniors fuller longer, and the protein can help to build muscle strength and reduce the risk of muscle loss. Making time for juicing and smoothie making for seniors over 60 doesn't have to be difficult. There are many easy and convenient options that can make it simple for seniors to make these healthy drinks. Blenders and juicers are available in various sizes, so seniors can find one that fits their needs and lifestyle.

Additionally, there are many pre-made smoothie and juice recipes available online, so seniors can find healthy and delicious options that are quick and easy to make. By making juicing and smoothie making part of their daily routine, seniors over 60 can benefit from the many health benefits these drinks provide. With a little bit of time and effort, seniors can easily incorporate juicing and smoothies into their daily routine and enjoy the many benefits that come with it.

How seniors can Plan and Preparing for Success

Planning and prepping for success is an important step for seniors over 60 who want to make juicing and smoothies part of their daily routine. Planning ahead can help to make the process of juicing and smoothie making easier and more efficient.

Prepping ingredients and equipment ahead of time can help to ensure that the process goes smoothly and that seniors have everything they need at the ready. One of the first steps seniors can take in planning and prepping for success is to buy the necessary tools and ingredients.

Investing in a good quality blender or juicer can help to make the process more efficient and enjoyable. Additionally, seniors should stock up on the necessary ingredients, such as fruits, vegetables, and other liquid ingredients like almond milk, coconut water, or Greek yogurt. Seniors should also plan out their recipes in advance. Deciding which recipes to make ahead of time can help to make the process easier and quicker.

This will also help to ensure that seniors have all of the necessary ingredients at hand. Additionally, seniors should take the time to wash and cut their ingredients, as this can help to make the process go faster.

By planning and prepping ahead of time, seniors over 60 can make the process of juicing and smoothie making easier and more efficient. Taking the time to plan and prep ahead of time can help to ensure that seniors have a successful juicing and smoothie making experience.

How seniors can Stay Motivated and Overcoming Obstacles

Staying motivated and overcoming obstacles is an important part of making juicing and smoothie making part of a daily routine for seniors over 60. While making these healthy drinks can be a great way for seniors to get in extra fruits and vegetables and to stay healthy, it can also be difficult to stay motivated and keep up with the routine. Fortunately, there are a few simple steps seniors can take to help them stay motivated and overcome any obstacles they may encounter.

First, seniors should set realistic goals for themselves. Making small, achievable goals can help to keep seniors motivated and on track. For example, seniors should try to make a certain number of smoothies or juices per week or per month. Setting goals like this can help seniors to stay motivated and reach their desired outcomes.

Secondly, seniors should find creative ways to make the process of juicing and smoothie making more enjoyable. Trying new recipes or adding unique ingredients can help to make the process more fun and interesting. Additionally, seniors should also look for ways to save time, such as prepping ingredients ahead of time or using a blender that allows for one-touch blending.

Finally, seniors should also not be afraid to ask for help if they need it. Having a friend or family member help with the process can make it much easier and more enjoyable.

Additionally, seniors can also look for online resources that can provide tips and advice on making juicing and smoothie making part of their daily routine.

By staying motivated and overcoming obstacles, seniors over 60 can make juicing and smoothies making part of their daily routine. Taking the time to set goals, make the process more enjoyable, and ask for help can help seniors to stay motivated and reach their desired outcomes.

How seniors can Incorporate Juicing and Smoothies into Social Settings

Incorporating juicing and smoothies into social settings can be a great way for seniors over 60 to enjoy the health benefits of these drinks while also spending time with friends and family. There are many creative ways for seniors to incorporate juicing and smoothies into social settings. One way seniors can incorporate juicing and smoothies into social settings is by hosting a juicing or smoothie bar party.

Seniors can invite their friends and family over and provide them with a variety of ingredients that they can use to make their own custom smoothies and juices. Additionally, seniors can also provide some pre-made recipes and offer helpful tips and advice on making the perfect smoothie or juice. Another way seniors can incorporate juicing and smoothies into social settings is by making them a part of a group exercise routine. Seniors can gather with their friends and family and go on a group walk or bike ride and then enjoy a healthy smoothie or juice afterwards.

This can be a great way to get in some exercise, socialize, and enjoy a healthy drink. Finally, seniors can also make juicing and smoothies a part of their regular meal routine. Instead of having a traditional breakfast or lunch, seniors can enjoy a smoothie or juice with their friends or family. This can be a great way for seniors to get in extra servings of fruits and vegetables and to enjoy quality time with their loved ones.

By incorporating juicing and smoothies into social settings, seniors over 60 can enjoy the health benefits of these drinks while also spending time with their friends and family.

Taking the time to get creative and find ways to make juicing and smoothie making part of social settings can be a great way for seniors to stay healthy and enjoy quality time with their loved ones.

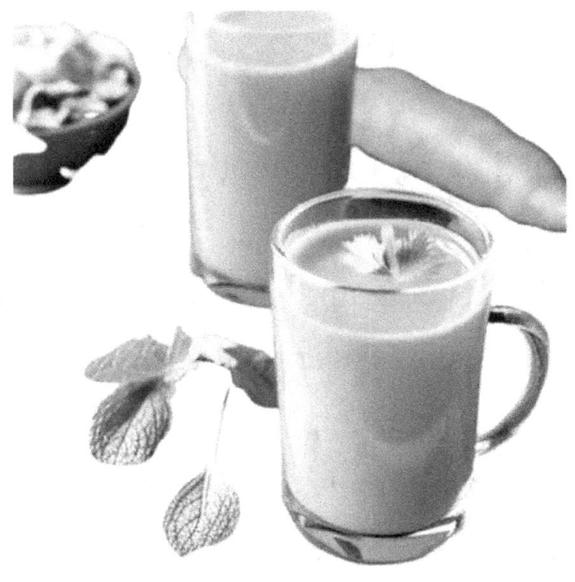

CONCLUSION

THE BENEFITS OF HEALTHY AGING THROUGH JUICING AND SMOOTHIES FOR MEN OVER 60

Making juicing and smoothies part of a daily routine can provide many benefits for men over 60. Juicing and smoothies can help to improve a man's overall physical and mental health and can help to maintain a healthy weight. Additionally, juicing and smoothies can provide men with essential vitamins, minerals, and other nutrients that are beneficial for overall health and vitality.

One of the main benefits of juicing and smoothies for men over 60 is **improved heart health.**

The fiber, vitamins, and minerals found in fruits and vegetables can help to reduce cholesterol levels and improve heart health. Additionally, the antioxidants found in these drinks can help to reduce inflammation and the risk of heart disease. Juicing and smoothies can also help men to maintain a healthy weight. Juicing and smoothies are a great way to get in extra servings of fruits and vegetables without the calories and fat that can come with more traditional meals.

Additionally, adding protein and fiber to one's diet can help to keep men fuller longer and can help to **build muscle strength** and reduce the risk of **muscle loss.**

Finally, juicing and smoothies can also help to **improve mental health**. The antioxidants found in these drinks can help to reduce inflammation and stress and can help to improve cognitive function and mental clarity.

Additionally, the vitamins and minerals found in these drinks can help to improve mood and overall well-being. By making juicing and smoothies part of a daily routine, men over 60 can benefit from the many health benefits these drinks provide. Taking the time to make time for juicing and smoothie making can help men to improve their physical and mental health and to maintain a healthy weight.

Review of the 62-Day Program

The 62-Day Healthy Aging Program outlined in this book "Healthy Aging through Juicing and Smoothies: A 62-Day Program for Men over 60" is an excellent program for men over 60 who want to make juicing and smoothies part of their daily routine. The program provides a comprehensive guide to incorporating these healthy drinks into one's diet and offers helpful tips and advice on making the process easier and more enjoyable.

The program is broken down into 6 weeks and provides detailed instructions on what to do each week. The program also provides a variety of delicious recipes for juices and smoothies, as well as helpful advice on how seniors can make time for juicing and smoothie making. Additionally, the program also offers helpful tips and advice on how to incorporate juicing and smoothies into social settings, how to stay motivated, and how to plan and prep for success.

Long-Term Benefits and Lifestyle Changes Making juicing and smoothie making part of a daily routine can provide many long-term benefits for men over 60. Incorporating these healthy drinks into one's diet can help to improve overall physical and mental health, as well as helping to maintain a healthy weight. Additionally, making juicing and smoothie making part of a daily routine can also help to **foster positive lifestyle changes** that can have lasting effects.

30 herbs and spices seniors above 60 can add to their smoothies and juice

- **Turmeric:** Contains curcumin, which has anti-inflammatory properties and may aid in reducing joint pain and improving cognitive function.
- **Cinnamon:** Can help regulate blood sugar levels, reduce inflammation, and improve brain function.
- **Ginger:** Can alleviate nausea, reduce inflammation, and improve digestion.
- **Cayenne pepper:** Contains capsaicin, which has anti-inflammatory properties and may

aid in reducing pain and improving heart health.

- **Black pepper:** Can improve digestion and increase the absorption of nutrients.

- **Rosemary:** Contains antioxidants and anti-inflammatory compounds that can improve brain function and reduce inflammation.

- **Oregano:** Has antibacterial and anti-inflammatory properties and may aid in reducing inflammation and improving gut health.

- **Thyme:** Contains antioxidants and anti-inflammatory compounds that can improve respiratory health and reduce inflammation.

- **Sage:** Can improve cognitive function, reduce inflammation, and enhance immune function.

- **Mint:** Can aid in digestion, reduce inflammation, and improve brain function.

- **Dandelion root:** Can aid in liver detoxification, reduce inflammation, and improve digestion.

- **Milk thistle:** Can aid in liver detoxification, reduce inflammation, and improve digestion.

- **Licorice root:** Can aid in reducing inflammation, improving digestion, and boosting immune function.

- **Astragalus:** Can enhance immune function and reduce inflammation.

- **Ginseng:** Can improve cognitive function, reduce inflammation, and enhance immune function.

- **Ginkgo biloba:** Can improve cognitive function, reduce inflammation, and enhance immune function.

- **Ashwagandha:** Can reduce stress, enhance immune function, and improve cognitive function.

- **Maca root:** Can improve energy levels, reduce inflammation, and enhance immune function.

- **Holy basil:** Can reduce stress, improve cognitive function, and enhance immune function.

- **Reishi mushroom:** Can enhance immune function, reduce

inflammation, and improve liver health.

- **Chaga mushroom:** Can enhance immune function, reduce inflammation, and improve gut health.

- **Lion's mane mushroom:** Can improve cognitive function, reduce inflammation, and enhance immune function.

- **Cordyceps mushroom:** Can improve energy levels, enhance immune function, and reduce inflammation.

- **Moringa:** Contains antioxidants, anti-inflammatory compounds, and may improve blood sugar levels.

- **Bee pollen:** Can improve immune function, reduce inflammation, and provide a source of protein.

- **Spirulina:** Can enhance immune function, reduce inflammation, and provide a source of protein.
- **Chlorella:** Can enhance immune function, reduce inflammation, and aid in detoxification.
- **Wheatgrass:** Contains antioxidants, anti-inflammatory compounds, and may aid in reducing inflammation and improving digestion.
- **Barley grass:** Contains antioxidants, anti-inflammatory compounds, and may aid in reducing inflammation and improving digestion.
- **Alfalfa:** Contains antioxidants, anti-inflammatory compounds, and may aid in reducing inflammation and improving bone health.

DAY PLANNER

Date: _______________

M   T   W   Th   F   Sa   Su

To Do

____

____

____

____

____

____

____

____

____

Priorities

Enthusiastic for

Appointments

____

____

____

Breakfast

Lunch

Dinner

Snack

Fitness

Mood

DAY PLANNER

Date:

M T W Th F Sa Su

To Do

Priorities

Enthusiastic for

Appointments

Breakfast

Lunch

Dinner

Snack

Fitness

Mood

DAY PLANNER

Date:

M   T   W   Th   F   Sa   Su

To Do

Priorities

Enthusiastic for

Appointments

Breakfast	Lunch	Dinner	Snack

Fitness	Mood

DAY PLANNER

Date: _______________

M T W Th F Sa Su

To Do

____
____
____
____
____
____
____
____
____
____
____
____

Priorities

Enthusiastic for

Appointments

____
____
____
____
____

Breakfast	Lunch	Dinner	Snack

Fitness

Mood

DAY PLANNER

Date:

M   T   W   Th   F   Sa   Su

To Do

Priorities

Enthusiastic for

Appointments

Breakfast

Lunch

Dinner

Snack

Fitness

Mood

DAY PLANNER

Date: _______________

M   T   W   Th   F   Sa   Su

To Do

Priorities

Enthusiastic for

Appointments

Breakfast

Lunch

Dinner

Snack

Fitness

Mood

DAY PLANNER

Date: _______________

M T W Th F Sa Su

To Do

____
____
____
____
____
____
____
____
____
____
____

Priorities

Enthusiastic for

Appointments

____
____
____
____

Breakfast

Lunch

Dinner

Snack

Fitness

Mood

DAY PLANNER

Date: ______________

M T W Th F Sa Su

To Do

Priorities

Enthusiastic for

Appointments

Breakfast

Lunch

Dinner

Snack

Fitness

Mood

DAY PLANNER

Date: _______________

M   T   W   Th   F   Sa   Su

To Do

Priorities

Enthusiastic for

Appointments

Breakfast	Lunch	Dinner	Snack

Fitness	Mood

DAY PLANNER

Date: _______________

M T W Th F Sa Su

To Do

Priorities

Enthusiastic for

Appointments

Breakfast

Lunch

Dinner

Snack

Fitness

Mood

DAY PLANNER

Date:

M   T   W   Th   F   Sa   Su

To Do

Priorities

Enthusiastic for

Appointments

Breakfast

Lunch

Dinner

Snack

Fitness

Mood

DAY PLANNER

M T W Th F Sa Su

To Do

Date:

Priorities

Enthusiastic for

Appointments

Breakfast

Lunch

Dinner

Snack

Fitness

Mood

DAY PLANNER

M   T   W   Th   F   Sa   Su

To Do

Date:

Priorities

Enthusiastic for

Appointments

Breakfast

Lunch

Dinner

Snack

Fitness

Mood

DAY PLANNER

Date: _______________

M T W Th F Sa Su

To Do

____

Priorities

Enthusiastic for

Appointments

| Breakfast | Lunch | Dinner | Snack |

| Fitness | Mood |

DAY PLANNER

Date:

M T W Th F Sa Su

To Do

Priorities

Enthusiastic for

Appointments

Breakfast

Lunch

Dinner

Snack

Fitness

Mood

DAY PLANNER

Date: _______________

M T W Th F Sa Su

To Do

____

____

____

____

____

____

____

____

____

____

Priorities

Enthusiastic for

Appointments

____

____

____

____

Breakfast	Lunch	Dinner	Snack

Fitness	Mood

www.ingramcontent.com/pod-product-compliance
Lightning Source LLC
Chambersburg PA
CBHW061025250726

48662CB00011B/1126